PCOS

DIET

COOKBOOK

FOR PREGNANCY

The Ultimate Guide with 20 Delicious & Quick Recipes for getting Pregnant and Boosting Fertility

Patricia Camire

CHECK OTHER BOOKS BY AUTHOR:

TABLE OF CONTENT

INTRODUCTION 5

CHAPTER ONE... 7

Navigating PCOS and Fertility: A Holistic Approach to
Pregnancy 7

Definition and Characteristics of PCOS........................ 7

PCOS and Fertility Challenges................................. 8

The Role of Diet in Enhancing Fertility with PCOS 8

Lifestyle Options for Fertility............................... 10

PCOS-Friendly Recipes for Pregnancy....................... 11

CHAPTER TWO 14

DELICIOUS AND EASY PCOS DIET RECIPES 14

1. Quinoa and Vegetable Stir Fry 14

2. Baked Lemon Herb Salmon.............................. 15

3. Berry and Greek Yogurt Parfait 16

4. Spinach and Feta Stuffed Chicken Breast 17

5. Quinoa Salad with Roasted Vegetables.................. 18

6. Sweet Potato and Chickpea Curry 20

7. Salmon and Asparagus Foil Packets 21

8. Lentil and Vegetable Stir-Fry 22

9. Greek Chicken Salad 23

10. Quinoa and Vegetable Stuffed Bell Peppers 24

11. Spinach and Mushroom Omelette............................ 26

12. Berry and Greek Yogurt Parfait 27

13. Grilled Lemon Herb Salmon................................... 28

14. Sweet Potato and Chickpea Curry 29

15. Avocado and Tomato Salad with Quinoa............... 30

16. Turkey and Quinoa Stuffed Bell Peppers............... 31

17. Spinach and Feta Omelette 32

18. Greek Yogurt Parfait with Berries 34

19. Salmon and Quinoa Bowl...................................... 34

20. Sweet Potato and Chickpea Curry 35

CONCLUSION 38

INTRODUCTION

In the enchanted realm of the "PCOS Diet Cookbook for Pregnancy," Emily embarked on an extraordinary gastronomic trip.

She wished for a comprehensive strategy to increasing fertility while suffering from PCOS. Patricia Camire's cookbook became her light of hope. Emily welcomed a renewed vibrancy as she devoured each dish, in addition to culinary treats.

The mornings began with the invigorating glow of a fertility-boosting smoothie, which set the tone for the day. Lunches were a symphony of colors and nutrition, with each component chosen to promote hormonal balance.

Emily felt the comfort of a nourished body as the fragrance of substantial dinners floated through her house, preparing her for the wonder of parenthood.

Each recipe, a work of art using fertility-friendly ingredients, evolved into a celebration of life. The cookbook was about more than simply cuisine; it was about realizing the possibilities in each mouthful.

Emily's PCOS struggle turned into a joyful quest for fertility, with the kitchen serving as a haven of well-being.

Emily not only learned how to make exquisite foods throughout her culinary expedition, but she also observed the tremendous influence of a well-planned diet on her reproductive quest.

Patricia Camire's cookbook was more than simply a compilation of dishes; it was a trigger for Emily's journey to parenthood.

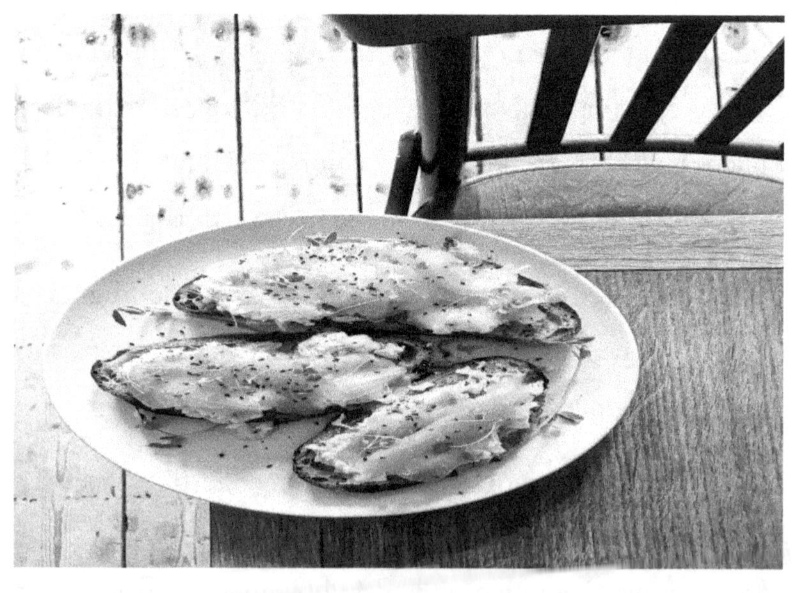

CHAPTER ONE

Navigating PCOS and Fertility: A Holistic Approach to Pregnancy

Polycystic Ovary Syndrome (PCOS) is a prevalent illness affecting women of reproductive age that causes hormonal abnormalities that can impair fertility. Understanding PCOS and its association with fertility is critical for people hoping to create a baby. This cookbook intends to shed light on the obstacles that women with PCOS may experience on their path to conception, as well as how a well-balanced diet may play an important part in improving fertility.

Definition and Characteristics of PCOS

Polycystic Ovary Syndrome is a complicated hormonal condition that presents in a variety of ways. Common symptoms include irregular menstrual cycles, ovarian cysts, and hormonal abnormalities.

These characteristics can make it difficult to conceive, therefore women with PCOS should seek early diagnosis and therapy.

PCOS and Fertility Challenges

PCOS presents unique reproductive issues, owing to irregular ovulation. Women with PCOS may have sporadic or nonexistent ovulation, which reduces their chances of conceiving naturally.

Understanding the relationship between PCOS and fertility is critical for people considering starting family.

The Role of Diet in Enhancing Fertility with PCOS

Nutrition is essential in preparing the body for pregnancy, particularly for women with PCOS. A diet high in critical nutrients can help balance hormones, increase insulin sensitivity, and provide an ideal environment for conception.

Balancing Hormones with PCOS-Friendly Foods

Certain meals can help women with PCOS achieve hormonal balance. Including whole grains, lean proteins, and healthy fats in your diet can help manage insulin levels and reduce inflammation, addressing some of the underlying reasons of reproductive issues.

Managing Weight for Fertility

Weight control is an important part of fertility for women with PCOS since excess weight can worsen hormone abnormalities.

A well-balanced diet, along with regular exercise, can help you achieve and maintain a healthy weight, which improves reproductive outcomes.

The Value of Vitamins and Minerals

Certain vitamins and minerals are vital for reproductive health. Folic acid, for example, is critical in avoiding neural tube abnormalities in the growing baby. A diet high in fruits, vegetables, and whole grains provides an appropriate quantity of these essential nutrients.

Supporting Ovulation with Nutrient-Dense Foods

Women with PCOS who want to conceive must optimize their ovulation. Leafy greens, berries, and fatty fish are nutrient-dense diets that can help with ovulation and fertility.

Understanding the body's unique demands during the menstrual cycle is critical for developing a fertility-friendly diet.

Lifestyle Options for Fertility

Stress Management and Fertility

Stress can harm reproductive health, and women with PCOS may be particularly vulnerable to its effects. Implementing stress-management practices, such as meditation and yoga, can improve general health and fertility.

Exercise and Fertility

Women with PCOS benefit from regular physical exercise because it helps with weight management, improves insulin sensitivity, and promotes general health.

Customized fitness programs can boost fertility and help to a healthier pregnancy.

PCOS-Friendly Recipes for Pregnancy

Preconception Nutrition

Prior to conception, preconception nutrition is critical. Recipes with fertility-boosting components such as whole grains, lean meats, and nutrient-dense veggies help provide the groundwork for a healthy pregnancy.

Breakfasts for Fertility

Breakfast selections that are both balanced and delicious and promote reproductive health might help to set a good tone for the day. Women with busy schedules benefit from quick and easy meals.

Lunches for Nourishment

Lunchtime meals are healthful for women with PCOS, delivering a balance of critical nutrients while appealing to a wide range of tastes and preferences.

Dinners to Improve Fertility

Evening meals emphasize taste and fertility, offering pleasant alternatives that are compatible with a PCOS-friendly diet.

Family-friendly dishes meet the nutritional demands of women with PCOS, making mealtime more pleasurable for everyone.

Snacks and Treats for Fertility

Snack and treat dishes provide guilt-free delights that satisfy the sweet and savory desires of PCOS patients. These dishes find a balance between flavor and nutrition. Managing PCOS and fertility on the way to conception necessitates a diverse strategy.

Understanding the complexities of PCOS, integrating a fertility-friendly diet, and living a healthy lifestyle can all help increase the odds of pregnancy.

The addition of PCOS-friendly pregnancy meals makes it easier and more fun for women with PCOS to start their parenthood journey.

Women may empower themselves on the wonderful journey of starting kids by embracing holistic practices and eating nutritious meals.

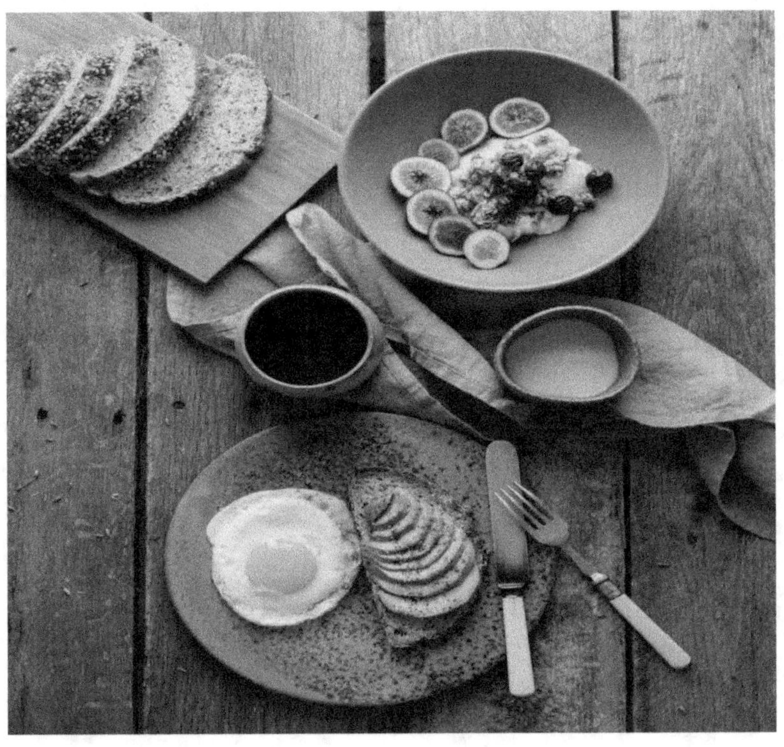

CHAPTER TWO

DELICIOUS AND EASY PCOS DIET RECIPES

1. Quinoa and Vegetable Stir Fry

Ingredients:

- 1 cup of quinoa

- 2 cups of mixed veggies (broccoli, bell peppers, carrots, and snap peas)

- One tablespoon of olive oil

- 2 garlic cloves, minced

- One tablespoon of low-sodium soy sauce

- One teaspoon of sesame oil

- Add Salt and pepper to taste

- ¼ cup of minced fresh cilantro (optional)

Prep Time: 25 minutes

Instructions:

1. Rinse the quinoa in cold water and cook according to package directions.

2. In a large pan, increase the olive oil temperature over medium heat. Pour the minced garlic and cook until fragrant.

3. Add the mixed veggies to the pan and stir-fry until soft and crisp.

4. In the pan, combine the cooked quinoa and veggies.

5. Drizzle soy sauce and sesame oil over the mixture. Add salt and pepper to bring out the flavor.

6. Toss everything until fully incorporated and cooked through.

7. If preferred, garnish with finely chopped cilantro.

2. Baked Lemon Herb Salmon

Ingredients:

- 4 salmon fillets

- 2 tablespoons of olive oil

- 1 lemon, juiced and zested

- 2 teaspoons of dried herbs (such as dill, thyme, or rosemary)

- Add Salt and pepper to taste

- Garnish with lemon slices

Prep Time: 20 minutes (plus marinating time)

Instructions:

1. Preheat the oven to 375°F (190°C).

2. In a small bowl, whisk together olive oil, lemon juice, lemon zest, dried herbs, salt, and pepper.

3. Place salmon fillets in a shallow dish and pour the marinade over them. Let it soak for minimum of 15 minutes.

4. Transfer the salmon fillets to a baking dish. Place a lemon slice on each fillet.

5. Bake in the preheated oven for 15-20 minutes or until the salmon peels effortlessly with a fork.

3. Berry and Greek Yogurt Parfait

Ingredients:

- 1 cup of Greek yogurt

- 1 cup of mixed berries (strawberries, blueberries, raspberries)

- 2 tablespoons of honey

- ¼ cup of granola

Prep Time: 10 minutes

Instructions:

1. In a glass or dish, place half of the Greek yogurt.

2. Arrange each mixed berries on top of the yogurt.

3. Drizzle 1 tablespoon honey over the berries.

4. Repeat layering with the remaining yogurt, berries, and honey.

5. For extra crunch, sprinkle granola over the top.

6. Serve immediately and savor this refreshing and healthy parfait.

4. Spinach and Feta Stuffed Chicken Breast

Ingredients:

- 4 boneless and skinless chicken breasts

- 2 cups of chopped fresh spinach,

- ½ cup of crumbled feta cheese

- 2 minced garlic cloves

- 1 tablespoon of olive oil

- Use 1 teaspoon of dried oregano

- Add Salt and pepper to taste

- Serve with Lemon wedges

Prep Time: 30 minutes

Instructions:

1. Preheat your oven to 375°F (190°C).

2. In a pan, cook the minced garlic in olive oil until fragrant. Add the chopped spinach and simmer until wilted. Remove from heat.

3. In a bowl, combine the sautéed spinach, crumbled feta cheese, dried oregano, salt, and pepper.

4. Cut a pocket in each chicken breast and fill with the spinach and feta mixture.

5. Using toothpicks, secure the pockets and arrange the packed chicken breasts in a baking dish.

6. Bake in the preheated oven for 25-30 minutes, or until the chicken is well done.

7. Serve lemon wedges on the side.

5. Quinoa Salad with Roasted Vegetables

Ingredients:

- 1 cup of quinoa

- 2 cups of mixed vegetables (zucchini, cherry tomatoes, bell peppers)

- 2 tablespoons of olive oil

- 1 teaspoon of dried thyme

- ¼ cup of chopped fresh parsley

- 1 lemon juice

- Add Salt and pepper to taste

Prep Time: 35 minutes

Instructions:

1. Cook the quinoa according to package directions and let it cool.

2. Preheat the oven to 400°F (200° C).

3. Mix the veggies with olive oil, dried thyme, salt, and pepper. Roast in the oven until tender.

4. In a large bowl, mix the cooked quinoa and roasted veggies.

5. Drizzle the salad with lemon juice and mix well.

6. Before serving, garnish with freshly cut parsley.

6. Sweet Potato and Chickpea Curry

Ingredients:

- 2 peeled and diced sweet potatoes

- 1 can (15 oz) of sapped and washed chickpeas,

- 1 finely chopped onion,

- 2 minced cloves garlic,

- 1 can (14 oz) of chopped tomatoes

- 1 can (14 oz) of coconut milk

- Two teaspoons of curry powder

- 1 teaspoon of turmeric

- Salt and pepper to taste

- Garnish with fresh cilantro

Prep Time: 40 minutes

Instructions:

1. Cook chopped onion and garlic in a large saucepan until softened.

2. Combine the chopped sweet potatoes, chickpeas, tomatoes, coconut milk, curry powder, turmeric, salt, and pepper.

3. Simmer the curry over medium heat until the sweet potatoes are cooked.

4. Adjust the flavor as needed and serve over rice.

5. Sprinkle with fresh cilantro before serving.

7. Salmon and Asparagus Foil Packets

Ingredients:

- 4 salmon fillets

- One bunch of trimmed asparagus

- Two teaspoons of olive oil

- 2 garlic cloves, minced

- One lemon, sliced

- Fresh dill as garnish

- Add Salt and pepper to taste

Prep Time: 25 minutes

Instructions:

1. Preheat oven to 400°F (200°C).

2. Place one salmon fillet on a piece of foil. Arrange the asparagus around the fish.

3. Drizzle olive oil on the fish and asparagus. Add crushed garlic, salt, and pepper.

4. Arrange lemon slices on top of each salmon fillet.

5. Seal the foil packets and bake in the preheated oven for 15-20 minutes, or until the salmon is well cooked.

6. Sprinkle with fresh dill before serving.

8. Lentil and Vegetable Stir-Fry

Ingredients:

- 1 cup of cooked dry lentils,

- 2 cups of mixed vegetables (broccoli, carrots, bell peppers)

- 3 tablespoons of soy sauce

- 2 tablespoons of sesame oil

- 1 tablespoon of rice vinegar

- 1 tablespoon of honey

- 2 chopped garlic cloves

- One teaspoon of grated ginger

- Green onions as garnish

Prep Time: 30 minutes

Instructions:

1. Stir-fry veggies in sesame oil until soft.

2. Add the cooked lentils to the skillet and continue to stir-fry.

3. In a small bowl, combine the soy sauce, rice vinegar, honey, chopped garlic, and grated ginger.

4. Pour the sauce over the lentil-vegetable mixture. Stir until evenly coated.

5. Continue cooking for a further 5 minutes, or until everything is well heated.

6. Before serving, garnish with thinly sliced green onion.

9. Greek Chicken Salad

Ingredients:

- 2 cups of cooked chicken breast (shredded)

- 2 cups of assorted salad greens

- 1 chopped cucumber,

- 1 cup of halved cherry tomatoes,

- ½ cup of crumbled feta cheese

- ¼ cup of pitted Kalamata olives,

- 2 tablespoons of olive oil

- 1 tablespoon of red wine vinegar

- 1 teaspoon of dried oregano

- Salt and pepper to taste

Prep Time: 20 minutes

Instructions:

1. In a large bowl, mix the shredded chicken, salad greens, sliced cucumber, cherry tomatoes, feta cheese, and Kalamata olives.

2. In a small dish, combine the olive oil, red wine vinegar, dried oregano, salt, and pepper.

3. Drizzle the salad with the dressing and toss to mix.

4. Serve immediately for a refreshing and filling salad.

10. Quinoa and Vegetable Stuffed Bell Peppers

Ingredients:

- 4 big halved bell peppers with seeds removed

- 1 cup of cooked quinoa,

- 1 cup of drained and rinsed black beans

- 1 cup of corn kernels

- 1 cup of cherry tomatoes, diced

- ½ cup of thinly minced red onion,

- 1 cup of shredded cheddar cheese

- 2 tablespoons of olive oil

- 1 teaspoon of cumin

- 1 teaspoon of chili powder

- Add Salt and pepper to taste

- Fresh cilantro as garnish

Prep Time: 40 minutes

Instructions:

1. Preheat your oven to 375°F (190°C).

2. In a large mixing bowl, add cooked quinoa, black beans, corn, cherry tomatoes, red onion, and shredded cheddar cheese.

3. Combine the olive oil, cumin, chili powder, salt, and pepper. Mix until well mixed.

4. Fill each bell pepper half with quinoa mixture.

5. Place the filled peppers on a baking tray and bake for 25–30 minutes, or until soft.

6. Before serving, garnish with chopped fresh cilantro.

11. Spinach and Mushroom Omelette

Ingredients:

- 3 big eggs

- 1 cup of chopped baby spinach,

- ½ cup of sliced mushrooms,

- ¼ cup of crumbled feta cheese,

- 1 tablespoon of olive oil

- Season with Salt and pepper to taste

- Garnish with fresh herbs, like parsley or chives

Prep Time: 15 minutes

Instructions:

1. In a mixing basin, whisk together the eggs until thoroughly combined. Season with salt and pepper.

2. Heat olive oil in a nonstick pan over medium heat.

3. Add the mushrooms and sauté until softened.

4. Add the chopped spinach to the pan and heat until wilted.

5. Pour the beaten eggs over the veggies and allow to set slightly around the edges.

6. Sprinkle crumbled feta cheese over the omelette and fold in half.

7. Cook for another 2-3 minutes, until the eggs are thoroughly cooked.

8. Prior to serving, garnish with fresh herbs.

12. Berry and Greek Yogurt Parfait

Ingredients:

- 1 cup Greek yogurt

- ½ cup of mixed berries, such as strawberries, blueberries, or raspberries

- ¼ cup of granola

- 1 tablespoon of honey

- Mint leaves as garnish

Prep Time: 10 minutes

Instructions:

1. In a glass or dish, layer Greek yogurt on the bottom.

2. Arrange each of mixed berries on top of the yogurt.

3. Sprinkle the granola over the fruit.

4. Drizzle the honey on the granola.

5. Repeat the layers until the glass or bowl is full.

6. Just before serving, garnish with fresh mint leaves.

13. Grilled Lemon Herb Salmon

Ingredients:

- 2 salmon fillets

- 2 tablespoons of olive oil

- 1 tablespoon of fresh lemon juice

- 1 teaspoon of dried dill

- 1 teaspoon of garlic powder

- Add Salt and pepper to taste

- Serve with lemon wedges

Prep Time: 20 minutes

Instructions:

1. Preheat grill to medium-high.

2. In a small bowl, combine the olive oil, lemon juice, dried dill, garlic powder, salt, and pepper.

3. Coat the salmon fillets with the lemon herb marinade.

4. Place the salmon on the prepared grill and cook for 4-5 minutes per side, or until readily flaked with a fork.

5. Serve with lemon wedges.

14. Sweet Potato and Chickpea Curry

Ingredients:

- 2 peeled and diced sweet potatoes

- 1 can (15 oz) of drained and washed chickpeas,

- 1 can (14 oz) of chopped tomatoes

- 1 finely cut onion,

- 2 minced cloves garlic,

- One tablespoon of curry powder

- 1 teaspoon of ground turmeric

- 1 teaspoon of cumin

- ½ teaspoon of paprika

- One cup of coconut milk

- Add Salt and pepper to taste

- Garnish with fresh cilantro

Prep Time: 30 minutes

Instructions:

1. Sauté onion and garlic in a large saucepan till tender.

2. Combine the sweet potatoes, chickpeas, chopped tomatoes, curry powder, turmeric, cumin, paprika, coconut milk, salt, and pepper.

3. Bring the mixture to a boil and cook for about 20-25 minutes, or until the sweet potatoes are cooked.

4. Adjust spice to taste.

5. Serve the stew over rice and top with fresh cilantro.

15. Avocado and Tomato Salad with Quinoa

Ingredients:

- 1 cup of cooked quinoa

- 1 diced avocado,

- 1 cup of cherry tomatoes (halved)

- 1 diced cucumber,

- ¼ cup of finely chopped red onion,

- 2 tablespoons of olive oil

- 1 tablespoon of balsamic vinegar

- Salt and pepper to taste

- Fresh basil leaves for garnish

Prep Time: 15 minutes

Instructions:

1. In a large bowl, mix cooked quinoa, diced avocado, cherry tomatoes, cucumber, and red onion.

2. In a small bowl, combine olive oil, balsamic vinegar, salt, and pepper.

3. Drizzle the dressing over the quinoa and toss to combine.

4. Just before serving, garnish with fresh basil leaves.

16. Turkey and Quinoa Stuffed Bell Peppers

Ingredients:

- 4 halved bell peppers with seeds removed

- 1 pound of ground turkey

- 1 cup of cooked quinoa

- 1 can (14 oz) of diced tomatoes (drained)

- 1 cup of black beans (drained and rinsed)

- 1 cup of corn kernels

- Add 1 teaspoon of cumin

- 1 teaspoon of chili powder

- Season with Salt and pepper to taste

- Top with shredded cheese (optional).

- Fresh cilantro as garnish

Prep Time: 40 minutes

Instructions:

1. Preheat oven to 375°F (190°C).

2. Cook ground turkey in a pan until browned. Drain any extra fat.

3. In a large mixing bowl, combine cooked turkey, quinoa, diced tomatoes, black beans, corn, cumin, chili powder, salt, and pepper.

4. Fill each bell pepper half with the turkey-quinoa mixture.

5. Put the filled peppers in a baking tray, cover with foil, and bake for 25 to 30 minutes.

6. If preferred, sprinkle with shredded cheese in the final 5 minutes of baking.

7. Before serving, garnish with chopped fresh cilantro.

17. Spinach and Feta Omelette

Ingredients:

- 3 eggs

- 1 cup of chopped fresh spinach,

- ¼ cup of crumbled feta cheese,

- ¼ cup of diced cherry tomatoes,

- ¼ cup of minced red bell pepper,

- One tablespoon of olive oil

- Add Salt and pepper to taste

- Garnish with fresh parsley

Prep Time: 15 minutes

Instructions:

1. In a bowl, mix together the eggs and season with salt and pepper.

2. Heat olive oil in a nonstick pan over medium heat.

3. Add the spinach, cherry tomatoes, and red bell pepper to the pan and sauté until softened.

4. Pour the whisked eggs onto the veggies in the skillet.

5. Sprinkle feta cheese over the top and heat until the edges are firm.

6. Carefully turn the omelette and cook until completely set.

7. Sprinkle with fresh parsley before serving.

18. Greek Yogurt Parfait with Berries

Ingredients:

- 1 cup of Greek yogurt

- ½ cup of mixed berries, such as strawberries, blueberries, or raspberries

- 2 tablespoons of honey

- ¼ cup of granola

Prep Time: 10 minutes

Instructions:

1. Layer Greek yogurt, mixed berries, and granola in a glass or dish.

2. Drizzle honey on top.

3. Repeat the layers.

4. Serve immediately as a refreshing, nutrient-dense parfait.

19. Salmon and Quinoa Bowl

Ingredients:

- 1 cup of cooked quinoa

- 1 flaked grilled or baked salmon fillet,

- 1 cup of steamed broccoli florets

- ½ avocado, sliced

- 1 tablespoon of olive oil

- Serve with lemon wedge

- Season with Salt and pepper for flavor

Prep Time: 20 minutes

Instructions:

1. In a bowl, combine cooked quinoa, flaked salmon, steamed broccoli, and sliced avocados.

2. Drizzle the olive oil over the bowl and season with salt and pepper.

3. Gently toss until combined.

4. Serve with lemon wedges on the side for a refreshing finish.

20. Sweet Potato and Chickpea Curry

Ingredients:

- 1 big peeled and diced sweet potato

- 1 can (15 oz) of drained and washed chickpeas

- 1 can (14 oz) of diced tomatoes

- 1 finely chopped onion,

- 2 minced garlic cloves

- One tablespoon of curry powder

- 1 teaspoon of ground cumin

- 1 teaspoon of ground coriander

- ½ teaspoon of turmeric

- Use 1 cup of vegetable broth

- 1 cup of spinach leaves

- Add Salt and pepper to taste

- Garnish with fresh cilantro

Prep Time: 30 minutes

Instructions:

1. In a large saucepan, sauté the chopped onion and garlic until tender.

2. Stir in curry powder, powdered cumin, ground coriander, and turmeric to coat the onion and garlic.

3. Add the diced sweet potato, chickpeas, tomatoes, and vegetable broth to the saucepan.

4. Bring the mixture to a simmer, then cook until the sweet potatoes are cooked.

5. Stir in the spinach leaves and simmer until wilted.

6. Add salt and pepper to taste.

7. Before serving, garnish with chopped fresh cilantro.

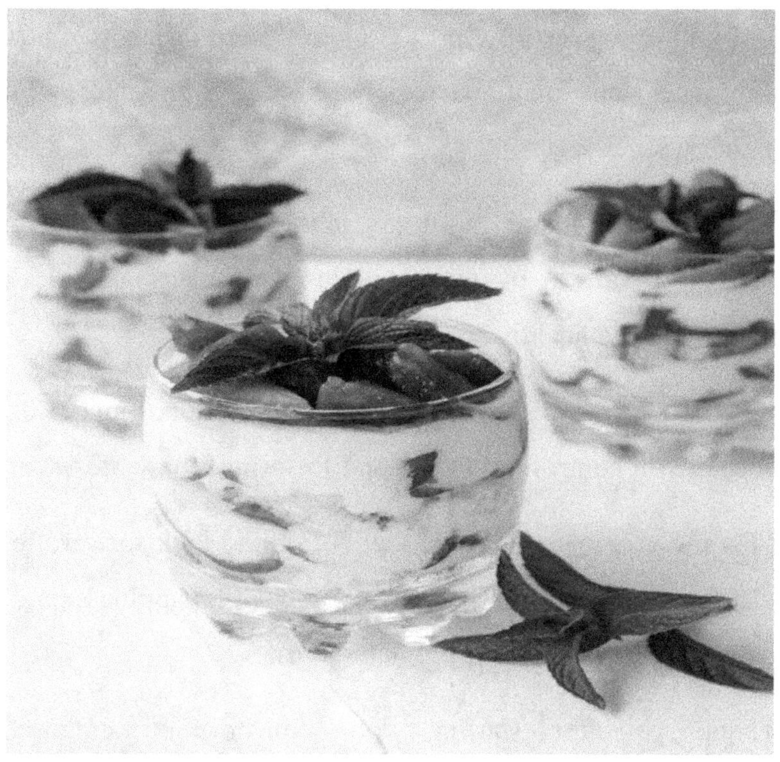

CONCLUSION

In concluding this PCOS Diet Cookbook for Pregnancy, we've embarked on a journey to empower women with PCOS to embrace a nourishing and delicious approach to pregnancy.

Understanding the significance of diet in controlling PCOS and improving fertility has led us to design dishes that not only meet nutritional demands but also celebrate the joy of eating well.

These dishes, created with care and deliberation, seek to deliver a variety of tastes while also assuring critical nutrients for a healthy pregnancy.

Remember that each dish represents the opportunity for harmony in controlling PCOS and fostering a new life.

May these recipes help you feel better and look forward to the wonderful trip ahead. I wish you health, happiness, and gastronomic joy on your pregnant journey.

Thank you for starting your transforming culinary adventure with the "PCOS Diet Cookbook for Pregnancy."

It has been a joy to guide you through the exquisite world of PCOS-friendly dishes designed particularly for the wonderful journey of pregnancy.

Your determination to nurture yourself and your little bundle of joy is admirable.

May these recipes bring happiness to your kitchen and health to your life.

As you taste each dish, keep in mind that you are doing more than simply eating; you are also nourishing the well-being of both you and your kid.

I wish you a happy and healthy pregnancy full of love, tastes, and moments of pure bliss.

Warm regards,

Patricia Camire

HAPPY COOKING!

www.ingramcontent.com/pod-product-compliance
Lightning Source LLC
Chambersburg PA
CBHW050753250726
48662CB00005B/2203